Pure Ann

A Collection of Poetry by Ann Jackson-Avery

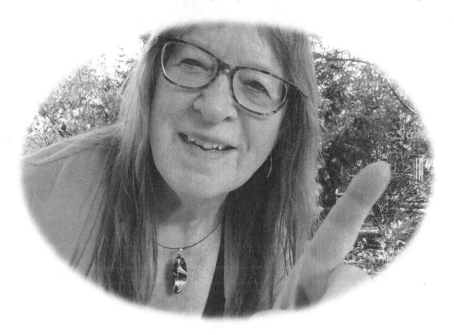

Volume One – Dance and Movement

Published by Friends & Family

Cover art created by Kim Long.
Cover design by Nita Alexander.

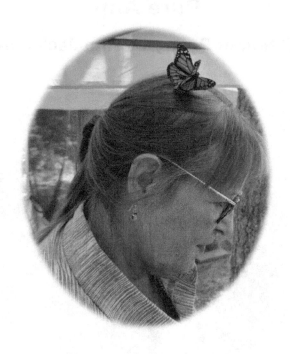

ISBN: 9798334882768

Imprint: Independently Published September 2024

About Ann

Ann Christine Jackson-Avery passed away on June 21, 2024, in Spokane, Washington, from an aggressive brain tumor at the age of 71.

Ann was a proud alumna of University (Cathedral) High School in San Diego and later earned a Bachelor of Science in Botany from San Diego State University. Her academic background paved the way for a diverse and impactful career. Ann held various positions in laboratory settings, including roles at Southwestern Community College and the Veterans Hospital Microbiology Department, where she met her beloved husband, Ken. The couple later moved to Spokane, where Ann continued her career at the Manito Gaiser Conservatory. She retired from the City of Spokane and subsequently took adjunct positions in horticulture and as a Brown Belt NIA dance instructor with the Community Colleges of Spokane (CCS). A significant chapter in Ann's life was her service as a Peace Corps volunteer in Tanzania in the mid-1980s, which enriched her perspective and deepened her commitment to community and global understanding.

Ann's hobbies reflected her love for the natural world and her creative spirit. Her passions for gardening, dance, and drumming were not just pastimes but a profound expression of her connection to nature and the arts. Her gardens were a testament to her skill and dedication, and her dance and drumming brought joy to many. She taught NIA dance for fifteen years and was an active part of the Spokane dance community.

Ann will be remembered for her generosity, her unwavering kindness, and her ability to inspire those around her. Her legacy will continue to influence and resonate with all who knew her. Ann's life was a beautiful, enduring garden she tended with love and now sustained in memory by those who loved her. (From her Obituary)

Introduction
by Kenneth Avery

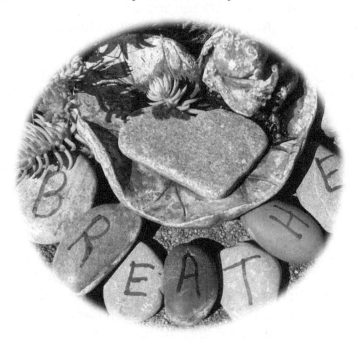

When I first came across this photo of yard art that can be commonly found in Ann's gardens and, in fact, everywhere Ann spent time being Ann, I said to myself out loud and without hesitation, "Pure Ann," and it brought me joy.

That same "earthy" spirituality was in her dance, poetry, art, gardening, music, meditation, nature, and every circle in which she participated. You will find that "breathing" is a thread that binds them all together and appears numerous times in this book. I see poetry in this photo.

It is as if some force in the universe guided me to this picture, at this time and in this context. Now I see it all around me, and I hope you will find some "Pure Ann" and feel her dancing, drumming, gardening, watching a butterfly, or simply making bread along with you.

Ann never had the chance to finish her desire to publish her poetry. She was writing it, dancing it, drumming it and baking it right up to the start of the ultimate journey she is now on.

She shared these poems after dance classes and meditative moments with friends. Many of the poems collected here are about dance, but not all. They are those she shared and identified with those moments.

They were unpublished until now. We do not know if what she wrote would have been what she would have published by her own hand. Some were handwritten and some in various digital formats. It is not for us to modify her art. So, we are publishing it as it was written or recorded. The beauty of this is that it remains "Pure Ann."

She had been writing poetry most of her life. As I uncovered more and more poems, pictures, drawings, and remembrances of her life and our shared life, the dance poetry that inspired this started to get overwhelmed by the volume of material, thus Volume One. It is the framework of near-future volumes that are already underway. Those will feature her poetry about family, friends, and nature.

"Ninakupenda sana"

Acknowledgements
by Kenneth Avery

All of Ann's friends and family deserve acknowledgement for the friendship and love they shared with her. Ann influenced them, and they influenced her. I would not be who I am without Ann, and therefore I am part of the circle as well.

We both received support and spiritual energy during her illness from so many of you that it is not possible to list everyone.

Thanks to those in Ann's dance circle that had the vision to keep Ann's poetry alive and in the process help all of us deal with our grief of losing a kindred spirit. I know it helped me immensely. Sincere gratitude to:

> Nita Alexander
> Debbie Brogan
> Kim Long
> Cat Macpherson
> Naomi Scher
> Kerry Wittsitt

Because of their efforts Ann can continue to dance in the hearts and spirits of others, she lives on.

This book will always make me cry, but they are tears of joy and bring to mind an image of "Pure Ann."

Table of Contents

A PEACEFUL RENEWAL

How can I accomplish renewal in myself?
How can I continue to grow in a more positive and
creative way?
        What will it take?

Perhaps getting rid of old thoughts and baggage from
my past.
Perhaps taking out that baggage
        and recycling it into something new,
                something healing for body and soul.

Perhaps getting rid of warring ways,
        my us vs. them mentality
                my conflicting thoughts and actions

Maybe I can "bury the hatchet" and let peace grow.
Maybe I can find new symbolic meaning
        in new thoughts and actions,
                and spread peaceful, strengthful gestures
                        like drum beats and heartbeats
Giving myself balance and renewal while practicing
self-love.

AJA March 2020

A PRAYER FOR PEACE

I detach from anything that seeks to separate.

Anything that says "us vs. them."

Anything that says "my way or the highway."

Anything that seeks to destroy, condemn, shame, or blame.

Instead, I choose unity.

I choose kindness, compassion.

I choose love.

-AJA, Date Unknown

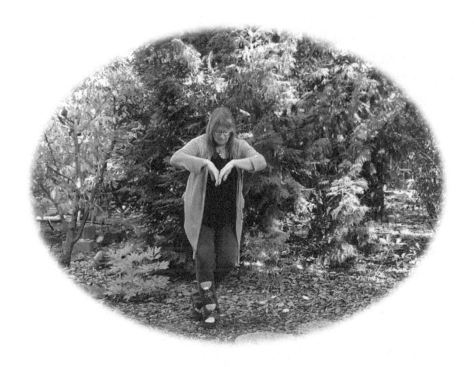

A Place I Go

There is a place I can go
when my body aches from the day to day,
here and there,
stopping and starting.

There is a place that I seek
when my mind is full
of lists and to-do
things spilling out
onto the desk.

There us a place I land
when emotions roil up
and threaten to take over
my very being.

My spirit beckons me there,
tho this place
in between the dark
and the light…

…inside the quiet,
the stillness
after the exhale
before the inhale
where my life hangs
in perfect balance
and I can rest
that perfect rest
of no worry
no hurry

just being with
myself
no judgement
no expectations
just
deep rest.

-AJA, Nov. 2022

AWARENESS: PAIN & PLEASURE

What does it mean to listen
to my conscious personal trainer
to help me become more aware
of my body? …Awareness…
Of pain, yes, I can feel the pain
in my feet & knees
hands & shoulders
head & heart.
And yes, I can adapt and adjust
my movements and my frame of mind
my viewpoint, my attitude
to make it feel better.
There will always be suffering,
but I must always continue
to ask myself…
What can I do to make it feel better?
And then, act on it.

But what else can I become aware of
in my being?
Pleasure, yes, I know what feels good,
what feels right.
I know what brings me joy.

Can I adapt that, adjust this,
and make my life even more joyful?

And what of those subtle aspects,
the energies, the sensations
of not just my Body, but also
my Mind, Emotions & Spirit?
What else am I missing
to bring my awareness into full view?

A prayer perhaps...
To my Body:
take care, nourish thyself & rest

To my Mind:
read, think, consider & rest

To my Emotions:
feel, allow, forgive, love & rest

To my Spirit: listen, make music and art, dance & rest

To my whole self:
breathe, move & mend

                                        -AJA, 11/30/2019

AWARENESS: TAKE TIME (LET YOUR BODY REST)

Let your awareness
take you on a journey
of your body,
your mind,
your emotions and spirit.

From your head to your toes,
from your outer extremities
to your deep, inner core…
ride the wave of your being.

Take time to sense your body, gently
move, stretch, squeeze and release.
Allow the pains and tightness
to melt into the earth.

Take time to perceive your mind, and its
various concerns, questions and worries.
Let them release to the wind
on the wings of peace.

Take time to feel your emotions, the highs
<u>and</u> the lows, of your everyday troubles;
the anger, sadness <u>and</u> excitements, as they
balance themselves into calmness.

Take time to sense your spirit; that unique
quality of you,
the inner essence of unconditional love.
Let it hold your body,
your mind and emotions.
Let it nurture and cultivate
the very best of you.

Take time…for awareness.

AJA, January 2021

BALANCE...

sense your balance in Body, Mind, Emotion, & Spirit

I look for balance_
(the yin and yang of life,)
everywhere I go_

from food cravings
to a healthy fullness_

from sleepiness
to wide awake_

from a foot weakness
to ankle strengthening_

from a shoulder tear
to muscle repair_

from headache
to full out bliss_

from a calm demeanor
to crazy animation_

I look to balance
my opposing energies_

I learned from a yoga teacher,
that balance is a point
we pass through
again and again_

I am never just at one point_

I am moving forward
or back_

looking one way
or another_

growing older
but thinking younger_

realizing my potential
while I ponder my past_

I am always on my way
somewhere_

                                    – AJA, February, 2023

BE A STAR

sense yourself as the stardust that you are
your part in the universe

yes, a tiny speck
but so much a part
of the wider whole

and just as important
just as intelligent
just as beautiful

now, open your hands wide
hold that universe
in the palms of your hands
and in the center of your heart

you are one with it
and it with you
in the center of your soul

release all to the universe

– AJA, Jan 12, 2020

BE SOFT IN YOUR PRACTICE

Be soft in your practice

but practice nonetheless.

Let the waters gently move you with joy.

Let them pulse and flow through your body

like dreamwalking through beauty.

Celebrate your practice,

your sacred life of dance

AJA, date unknown

Be Still

Let your body sink
into the earth,
sensing the primal rhythms,
connecting
with your heart beat,
your rhythmic breath,
your pulse.

Be Quiet

Let your mind's thoughts
swirl and flow and drift
until they are silent,
resting,
recovering,
restoring your peace.

Be Healed

Let your emotions
find equilibrium.
Balance the highs and lows
to allow stress and strain
to melt...
and healing begin.

Be Devoted

To your own self,
to your growth and
quest for understanding,
to your kindness and compassion
for yourself and all others

What else are we here for?

— AJA, October, 2022

BODY SENSATIONS

My Body senses many things.
Hot, cold, rain and blowing dust,
pain and pleasure,
sadness and joy.
These help me live my life
and mend myself,
body, mind, emotion and spirit.

These sensations give me energy
in the stretch of an early morning
wake-up,
reaching down for my slippers,
the tingly, warm feel of Flexibility,
opening and lengthening,
my energy moving outward.

My Body notices Agility,
that sense of easy start and stop,
as when I brush my teeth,
quick up, down and around motions,
or chopping veggies for dinner,
or running to quickly close the gate,
so the wind doesn't slam it shut.

My Body perceives Mobility
when walking the garden,
moving from weed to weed,
flower to flower,
swirling around to notice
birds here and there,
looking for the perfect spot

to sit or stand…in Stability…
the harmony and peace,
my energy centered,
but ready for action…if needed.

My Body is aware
of when my Strength energy
is sapped.
But I can also feel my Strength
building when I work in the garden,
or lift weights, or dance,
containing and sustaining my power.

My Body has power…
the power to sense it's needs,
and using those energy sensations,
flexibility, agility, mobility and strength.
I have the power of endurance,
patience and renewal,
and the power to heal myself,
from the inside out.

AJA, Spring 2022

BREATH MEDITATION

Breathe in
Breathe out
Belly rise
      Belly sink
Expanding lungs
      Releasing heart
In and out
      In and out.

Let sound flow in
      Emotions rush out
Sense them
      Acknowledge them
Allow them
      They are yours.
Let quiet enfold
      Calming, nurturing

Diminishing pain
      Releasing worry
I am free
      Right now.

Waves of light
>And quiet dark
Rain and sun
>Play and rest
Heart beating
>Blood pumping
Every day
>Is another chance
To live
>And breathe.

In and out
>In and out
>>In and out

(Oct. 2012)

BREATHE IN

…relaxation into your body
Deep release…calm…letting go

Breathe in

deep into your belly
into your back
and from your head
to your toes & back again.

Breathe in

peace & serenity
…into your mind
allowing tranquility,
allowing freedom from worry
and care

Breathe in

strength… to your heart
let your emotions
be brave
in your search for
harmony & balance.

Breathe in

the wholeness of you
allow your unique <u>spirit</u>,
full of wonder & creativity
to shine through
and infuse
your everyday life.

Breathe in

healing
that sense of
happiness & well-being
joy & contentment,
healing
to all the cells of your body,
healing, into the deep recesses
of your mind,

healing,
into the everyday peaks & valleys
of your emotions,
and into your ever-present,
loving spirit,

Breathe…Breathe…Breathe

-AJA, 2021-2023

BREATHE WITH...

Breathe with your Body
Use its gifts to sense
your lungs, your belly,
your fingers and toes.
sense the relaxation…wash over you like waves

on the sand as you breathe.

Breathe with your Mind.
See your cluttered thoughts
flutter and float by
like clouds in the sky
as you begin to ease your
viewpoints, imaginings
and assumptions.

Breathe with your Emotions.
Feel the hot sun of intensity,
your passions, reactions
and responses, soften with
each inhale and exhale
to encourage and support
your healing.
Honor all your Emotions;
but remember,
if you don't share your inner joys they will

be missed by the world.

Breathe with your Spirit.
Let that sense of your uniqueness
show you the beauty of life;
the beauty of water & earth,
fire & air…laughter & tears
all of which you are part…
life in all its strangeness,
challenges and questions,
some of which
you have no control.

Breathe…with your own mantra.
let your breath fill you with love
for yourself
and everything around you
for we are here to experience
the joy and pains of life,
in all those unique ways.

There is still so much beauty;
hold on to it.
You have the power,
over your own body,
your own emotions,
your own mind and heart.
Breathe with it.
Heal with it.

-AJA, Sept2021/May 2022

CLOSE YOUR EYES & HOLD YOUR HEART

Close your eyes
and hold on to your heart.

Sense the pulse
of your heart beatin
with the silence pouring
over your mind…

Now widen your circle of
awareness
and sense the pulse
of the heart beat
of others in the circle
around you…

Widen again to your
awareness of the earth
and the pulse of life
coming from earth…
…new shoots pulsing
up from the soil
…new green leaves pushing
their way open to the sun.

Flowers bursting forth,
their colors dazzling.
Our eyes and hearts
beating to their botanical pulses
and flowing
to the rhythm of life.
It belongs to us all…as we move
into our own dance

AJA, April 2019

COMING BACK

Coming back to you now
To this body
Sensing hands and feet
Hips and shoulders
Head and heart

I feel a twinge
an evolution
a learning that has taken place
a shift in my body
and its knowledge of pain
and pleasure
what feels wrong
what feels right
a year of living dangerously
will do that
giving me another perspective
new insight
An acceptance
of what cannot change
a chance, to change what I can and, a reminder
to breathe, just breathe
take care of what;s most important today-
moment to moment

So grateful now
for the time we have together
so grateful for
this body
especially the twinges, the shifting
the evolution
the learning
the knowledge that I can heal myself
do the best I can
for myself
and for others all around me

It's all coming back
to me now

AJA Summer 2021

CONNECT TO THE WATER

Sense your body rest into the Earth.
Breathe in the damp air.
Feel the sweat on your skin,
and the exchange of moist air
from your breath...
The atmosphere inside your body,
to the outside air around you.

Breathe and feel now,
the fluid pumping
in your connective tissues,
your joints, your veins and arteries,
from your Heart
all throughout your body.
Heart pumping, fluid flowing
from inside to out.

Now see in your mind
the River flowing nearby.
Breathe in its humidity.
See it flowing, tumbling, rolling,
sometimes slowly, sometimes wildly
nourishing our land, and us.
As the river flows on,

see it feeding creeks as it moves
and winds its way, all the way
to the Sea.

And as you imagine the riverwater
finding its way to the Ocean,
with Sun shining down,
sense the evaporation and formation
of clouds,
their movement across the Sky,
the water finally falling,
raining back onto the Earth
to nurture it once again.

Sense now,
your connection to this flow,
this water of Earth
and the water of your body,
from your body to the Earth and back,
as you breathe, sweat,
flow and replenish.
Water is Life.
Flow with its aliveness.

– AJA, March 2021

DANCE IS...TRIBAL

Dance is...tribal
                but inclusive
It is sacred.
It is vulnerable.
It is aloneness and togetherness.
It is magical and transformative.
It is sweaty energy.
It is difficult.
It is easy.
It is ecstatic.
It is attitude.
It is joyful and playful.
It is sorrowful and contemplative.
It is in my blood.
It is in my bones.
It is in my heart.
It is...dance.

-AJA, Date Unknown

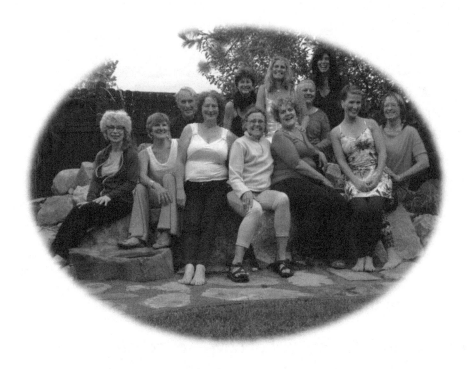

EMOTIONAL ENERGY

The sensation of the push and pull of LIfe.

The sensation of
feelings…swirling
around my head
and heart, inviting
me this
way…forcing me
that way. What do
I feel
today…moment to
moment?
How will I feel tomorrow?

What exactly is driving my emotions?

Love and Fear.

These are the root emotional choices I have.

I can choose to act…out of Love…or act out of Fear.

These are the basics…and I cannot live without either
one of them.

I can choose to act out of
Fear…wearing my mask
and avoiding crowds, to
protect my Self from
grave viral illness.

Or, I can choose
to act out of
Love…for my
Self and Others,
doing those very
same actions.

It is a matter of perception.
We are born with innate Love and Fear sensations and responses.
It is how we have survived on this earth.
Fear gives us clues to our safety, or lack thereof.
We can choose to act with Love about those things we Fear.
We can choose to act with Peace of mind,
to walk through our daily journey…our daily trial,
with Love in our hearts…even when Fear pushes or pulls us.
We have the choice.

AJA Feb 2021

EVEN AFTER A TREE DIES

Even after a tree dies
its tiny, upper branches leave
a lovely twisted impression
of its former life
a tapestry of phloem and xylem
once flowing and vibrant
now just a dream of what once was

But oh, if we are lucky
it also leaves behind stout, lower limbs
of hard wood standing firm
for as long as the elements will allow
a place for bird and insect homes
mosses, lichens
and endless wonderment

And so it is with us
these human forms
reaching high to the heavens
yet still rooted to the earth
We suffer so many traumas
in this one life…

The loss of childhood
and the myths of our innocence,
the demise of our loved ones
…and of our former selves
as we seek transformation

We know not how we shall become
but we know we need rebirth
as clearly as a meadowlark
sings his spring song
from a twisted branch

Renew your soul, and your earth
For as long as the elements will allow

AJA April 2019

FACE OF THE EARTH

Gaze upon the sky,
clouds driving and lifting,
giving a drop or ten
of heaven's tears, to
wash the cobwebs from our eyes
so we can see with new vision.

Gaze upon the earth,
the greens returning,
flowers renewing,
their colorful bells and faces
gazing back at us.

They will always come,
even in war,
even in dark and polluted skies,
reminding us to
think
and act for the good of all.

The face of earth
watches us,
warns us
at every turn,
every storm,
every fire,
every movement of Earth
tells us
we are not in charge.

Will we finally see,
listen and think
to take care of our Mother,
And all her beauty?

We are her life blood,
we have the power
to change, to heal,
to free ourselves
from our own greed
and hate
for a better fate on the Earth.

Open your eyes
and see,
as if a new born babe
with beginners mind.

AJA, For Earth Day 2023

FIND YOUR STRENGTH

(Original by AJA for 3-3-2019 Ecstatic Dance)

It took me a long time to Regain my Self
after my Father passed 36 years ago (tomorrow)
It drained me of my Happiness… my Hope… and my
Strength

and although I've lost many others
over these 30-some years……it never gets easier
The question still comes…why…..why the pain &
suffering, again & again
but I know I am Not Alone…we share this connection.

How DO we Recover our Selves again…
        when we know we must face the inevitable Trials
of Life
How do we Repair our Hope and Happiness
How do we Find our Strength again?

Find it…...Deep in your Breath
            Deep in your Heart
            Deep in your Soul…..for you are stronger
        than you think

Find your Strength
        In the Smile of a Stranger
        and the Hug of a Friend
        In the Love & Connection of your Community

Find it ....in letting out the Anger & Pain & Frustrations
from time to time
        ....and in Loving and Caring, and Forgiving Your
Self & Others

Find your Strength
        In your Ability to get up every day
        And walk your Dog....and feed your Cat....and
pet your Fish
Find it in the Wind and Birdsong outside your window
        ...and in the patterns of nature all around you

Find your Strength
        In your integrity, and in service to others
        And in your need to sometimes take a mental-
health day for Your Self

Find your Strength in Music & Silence.... in your
Stillness...and in Your Dance

Find it in letting go..........the Balance of Life is ever-
present

Find Your Strength (for Nia Martial Arts...)

There are so many trials in life, so much suffering
that can sap our strength,
cause us to lose faith, lose hope, lose perspective.

But we do have a choice on how to respond.
How can we recover ourselves again
when we know we must face the inevitable trials of
life?
How do we repair our hope and happiness, and find
our strength again?

Find it…deep in your breath…deep in your
heart…deep in your soul…
for you are stronger than you think.

Find strength in your body, your mind and emotions,
and in your spirit.

Find your strength in your ability to move,
in your ability to <u>block</u> what's not necessary,
to <u>strike</u> at the heart of your adversities,
to <u>punch</u> a hole in your doubts; to <u>kick</u> down the door
of fear.

Find your strength in the smile of a stranger
and the hug of a friend, in the love and connection of
community.

Find it in letting out the anger and frustrations from
time to time,
and in loving and caring, and forgiving your self and
others.

Find your strength in your ability to get up every day,
and walk your dog, feed your cat, and pet your fish.
Find it in the wind and birdsong outside your window,
and in the patterns of nature all around you.

Find strength in your integrity, and in service to others,
and in your need to sometimes take a mental-health
day for your self.

Find your strength in music and silence, in stillness
and in your dance.
Find it in letting go…
The balance of life is ever-present.

-AJA, Revised Spring, 2022

FORM & FREEDOM OF MA

I learn the dance…step by step
stance by stance
the routine of move here, then there
my feet follow the rhythm
of the music
the masculine drum beat
that Yang energy
leading the way of the form
sensing Taekwondo perhaps
the strength and agility of
blocks, kicks, punches, strikes
powerful strength and precision
from My body!

I move the dance…
feeling more confident
feeling freedom, feeling emotions
highs & lows from the music
the feminine song, Yin energy
melodically guiding my path
while the dance moves me
with the energy of Tai Chi perhaps
energy flowing slowly
from deep within
sensing that energy ball
balancing mobility with stability
balancing Yin & Yang.

I energize the dance…
full throttle, feet & hands
moving in sync, or
chaotically innovating
perhaps the spiral blending
of Aikido, harmonious motion
high, low, fast, slow
merging, melding, mending my soul.

It is my choice
having both the form to guide me
and the freedom to explore…
the push-pull of flexibility & mobility
toward or away from the earth
open & close my joints
squeeze & release my muscles

The yin & yang of form & freedom
at my disposal, blended & balanced.
It is my birthright to dance this way.
It is my birthright
to spontaneous creativity.

-AJA, Spring/Summer, 2021

HEAL LEAD

I start with my feet
their tender bunions
and crooked toes.
I flex my ankles
up and down,
point my toes
forward and back.
That feels good
to sense their flexibility
and mobility.
They still get me where I'm going
even with their flatness and bumps!
Their movements are healing
and they are mine.

I open my feet out
bending my knees to follow my toes
into different stances
from closed to open,
"A" to sumo,
sensing stability in bow
and cat stance.
I know I can increase
that sense of stability
and strength
in my muscles and joints
by playing with moving
back and forth, gently

from one stance to another.
A healing remedy for stiffness
and ache.

My stances become steps
to increase my agility,
the quick start and stop
as I cross front, cha cha cha,
as I step around my body's clock,
as I kick in all directions
and sweep my knee
to open my hips.

I sense all that I can do
to strengthen my lower extremities,
from my heel lead to my back kick,
their movements are healing
and they are mine.

-AJA, May 2021

I AWAIT THE SPRING

The crisp, cold, sunny, dry air
tells me NO!
Not yet!
But I don't care.

I await the Earth's crust
breaking open.
Crocus and snowdrops will
push up their smooth green leaves;
flowers to sing in the sun.
I await the Spring.
Bitter winds blowing bits
of white crystals,
taunting my face
cooling my desires

But I know if I wish hard enough
Spring rains will
warm the branches of rhody
and forsythia,
pushing buds to open,
bright yellow and purple,
fierce against cool showers

I await the Spring,
for I know it will
bring new days
warmer days
singing days
dancing days
days of growth
and transformation
and the opportunity
for hope.

-AJA 1/18/2021

ILLNESS

Illness knocks me for a loop
when I least expect it.
Slaps me in the face and chest
bringing me to my knees.
I'm not in charge.
Oh well.
Another chest cold
to cough out
while holding my painful head.
I really must go to the doctor.
Take care of myself.
Stop pushing so hard and fast.
Slow down.
Listen to my body.
Listen to the wind and rain.
Listen to my mind
Listen to the silent snow.
Listen to my heart,
to its rhythm and flow.
Listen to my spirit say:
Slow down,
Take care.

-AJA, Nov 2022

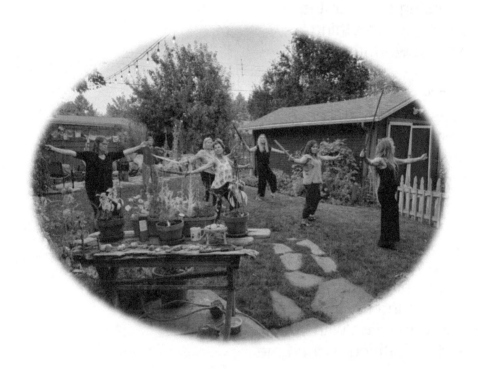

ILLUMINANCE

Sun rising
sheer gleaming brightness
emanating brilliant rays
fingers of light
reaching out
radiating the star it is
touching everything
with its warmth

Tears of joy
at its glowing brilliance
warming my skin
my heart
my spirit
with its golden clarity

Oh, if only
my own light
could shine as bright
illuminating my inner being
my connection with you
and everything around me

My body would dance
my heart would sing
my spirit would soar
into universal clarity itself
sharing the knowledge
of all that is
and what could be

Let's take a long, warm look
at that sunlight
and all of its gifts

AJA, Nov. 2022

INTO, ONTO, WITH

Sense your body in stillness.
Feel the coolness
of the floor beneath
and the air movement above.
Split into yourself
and take it all in for a moment
as you rest.

Slowly open your eyes.
Allow your body to turn onto one side
and let your open eyes gaze
upon another in the room.
Direct your attention 100%
on that one person
as we all begin to slowly move.
Perhaps swaying
or maybe reaching a hand up
or bending a knee. You choose.
Perhaps shifting to the other side.
Let yourself ellipt onto that person,
matching their moves
in your own way.

Finally, bring half of your attention
back to yourself
while still attending to the other.
"50/50" blending your attention
to self and other
as you continue moving up
to a sitting position, still moving
and shifting your body,
dynamically guiding your hands
up and out, consciously moving
your head from side to side.

Gradually bring your attention
back to your own self, 100%, moving
and preparing to rise
from the floor
and begin your Body Gratitude Walk.

Sensing body.
Sensing breath.
Thank you, Body.
I feel better

– AJA, November 10, 2021
(adapted from NiaNow.com)

LET YOUR MIND RELAX

Let go of the days' anxieties
    and any thought of tomorrows' concerns
Let your mind release now…your tension…your
fears…your worries
Let it all go…..and let your mind be filled with
calm………………………………………
Now gently, consider the two parts of your **brain** inside
your head
    the left and the right hemispheres…just notice
them
    the physical place where the mind might reside
The left side providing logic, fact-based, analytical
thinking
The right side giving artistic intuition, visualization, and
creative thinking
The two sides connected together by bundles of
nerves
    chemical and electrical activity
    efficiently complimenting and coordinating with
each other
    into the miracle that is your brain
Now, consider your **mind**
    Does it just reside inside your brain inside your
head?
    Or, can it also be found in your heart and your
gut
    as well as your head?
Do you not feel the empty sadness in your heart or gut
    when you <u>know</u> you have lost a loved one?

Do you not feel the enormous wonder of nature all throughout your body
at the sight of a glorious sunset on a beach? Or in the face of a flower.
The beautiful, miraculous mind.
Your mental energy produces your reasoning, feelings, memories, imagination
and indeed your personality.
Mental energy with all its intricate and infinite variations
makes each of us unique, no matter where the mind resides.

-AJA, Feb, 2021

LIFE FORCE

What keeps me going…day to day…hour to
hour…moment to moment?
What moves my Life Force along?
What shapes my Vitality…my quest for continuing…my
drive to be & be seen?
It's innate, I know…inherent…intrinsic…it's in my
nature, to be.
How then, can I optimize my Life Force Energy?
How then, can I increase, circulate and utilize this
Energy?
Here's how:
By consciously managing my physical energy,
my body's battery, with its + and - sensations.
By taking the right steps and actions
to invest in my now and future body.
By eating right…sleeping right…moving
right…breathing right.
By striving for positive thoughts and intentions.
By acting ethically…and doing my best...for me.
My Life Force then, just might help others around me

AJA , Jan. 29, 2021

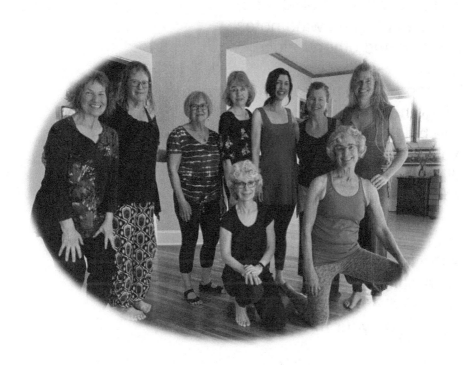

LISTENING (SILENCE & SOUND)

I sense you even before you start,
perhaps with percussive
tink-tinks
or boom-booms;
perhaps with flute or strings;
a voice of high flowing notes
ethereal and otherworldly.

Perhaps your sounds come
altogether, at once,
one big bang of sounds,
waves and waves of music
filling the air around me.
What joy in the sounds!

But most interesting
is the feeling, that longing;
the emotion of our meaning,
or at least
my take on your meaning.

How does it make me feel?
Can I name it?
And more importantly,
do I allow myself
to express that feeling
in my body? In my dance?
Oh Music!
It is so good to feel,
the sorrow and the joy.
We can all relate.

And what of the silence?
It can happen all around too,
maybe in fits and starts,
hidden between the phrases.
If only I would listen,
and sense that stillness, quiet
in the air.

There are messages in the music,
and the stillness,
only my body can feel,
only my mind can name,
only my spirit can use
for my healing.

– AJA, Oct. 2022

MY STRENGTH (MA & FAMSS)

Tai Chi – The Slow Dance (Shifting Flow of Energy)
Taekwondo – The Dance of Precision (BKPSC)
Aikido – The Dance of Harmonious Spherical
Motion (Spirals)

When I think of the **Martial Arts**
I think of **Strength**
and its relationship with
Flexibility
Agility
Mobility
and **Stability** (or FAMSS)

My strength is fluid & mobile
flowing from the inside out
sometimes showing stability
as slow moving energy
shifting from one space to another
high to low and side to side

Sometimes my strength comes
in the quick, firm agility movements
of blocks & kicks
punches & strikes & chops
Making my wishes known
with the precision of a cat

My strength is also revealed
in the spiraling of a turn
a shoulder or a hip opening
using mobility & flexibility
adapting to a change in
circumstance
blending with an opposing force
deflecting & modifying that force
a transformation in the dance

Strength comes in many forms
has many qualities
it is vital
powerful
courageous
as well as having the capacity
for endurance, patience
and renewal

My strength is fluid & flexible
agile & mobile
giving me stability
from the inside out

...AJA, 4/19/21

MEDITATION

now, you are
now, you can breathe
it is not yesterday
it's not tomorrow yet
so breathe
just breathe

listen to your breath
hear your heart
your emotions
your mind
your spine
your limbs, your lovely bones

listen to your smile
your laughter
your silly jokes
your dreams
and your loves

think
what else
are the good things about you?
speak them
hear them
be inspired by them
be inspired by the lovely beings
who gave you life
and love
and silly jokes

just breathe
be inspired by your own being

AJA, Fall 2023

Breathe in
Breathe out
Belly rise
   Belly sink
Expanding lungs
   Releasing heart
In and out
   In and out.

Let sound flow in
   Emotions rush out
Sense them
   Acknowledge them
Allow them
   They are yours.
Let quiet enfold
   Calming, nurturing
Diminishing pain
   Releasing worry
I am free
   Right now.

Waves of light
  And quiet dark
Rain and sun
  Play and rest
Heart beating
  Blood pumping
Every day
  Is another chance
To live
  And breathe.

In and out
  In and out
    In and out.

AJA, Oct 2012

MOVE FORWARD

There is no need
to relive the suffering.
Let it pass as experience
and insight gained.

Move forward,
in your pursuit
of joy and inner harmony.

Days of grief and discomfort
will always come,
for they may still hold
knowledge to be gained.

But your gifts
your wisdom,
and your practice
will see you through.

Peace resides within you.
Slow down
and let it heal you.

-AJA, October 2022

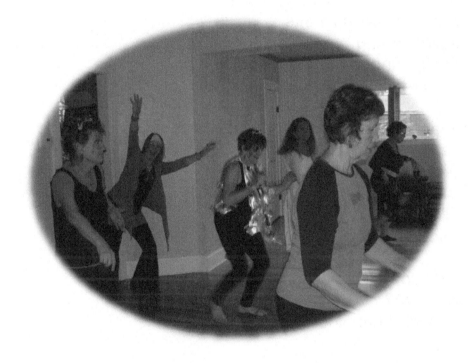

MY EVERYDAY NEEDS

What does my body need
right now?
...in my bones, my joints,
my muscles
sensing long bones and short
sensing spiraling joints
circling strong
sensing finger muscles gripping
then radiating out in all directions

What does my mind need
right now?
...quiet and calm
from the chaos all around me
stillness and deep rest
to soothe and heal

What do my emotions need
right now?
...outward happiness
and inner joy
to reign over sadness
and pain
deep peace within
to keep me whole

And what of my spirit?
Only I can know that
for it is deeply personal
and profound
and always striving
to his highest consciousness
All of this I need right now
for healing
and for every day forward

– AJA, October 2022

My "Mystery" Symbology (simplified)

In this routine, the image that arises for me is that
I am on a journey.
A simple journey as an animal (white pelican
perhaps?)
looking for water.

There are obstacles along the way that I must face.
A snake perhaps, or a tiger.
Boulders that must be broken apart,
cliffs to fly over, seeking water.

Now and agin I find a pool where I can refresh myself
along with all
the other animals and plants.

(on a deeper level)
* I strive to sense myself as one of the many in this
world, and beyond,
all living our lives as best we can.

* That connection to other things (both living and non-
living)
        keeps me whole, and contributes to my own
well-being.

* So this is an invitation to sense this in your own way,
finding your own symbology.

AJA, 7//19/2022

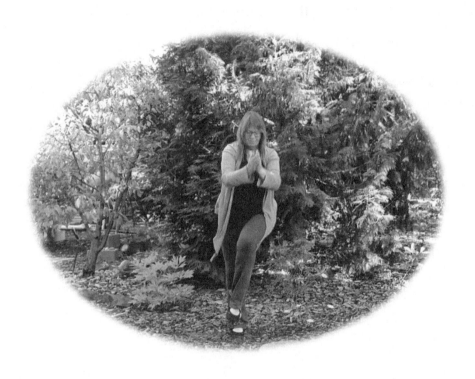

MY RELATIONSHIP WITH THE POWER OF TWO

Do I speak now,
Or listen?
What is needed at this precise
Moment?
I have the power in this relationship To

choose between the two.

But when my mind
Wanders and wonders,
What to do
What to say next,
I miss the opportunity
To listen
And hear the other,
Or silence
For the message that perhaps
Will change my Life.

Do I listen
Or do I speak?

For now, maybe
A quiet mind
Would give me
The blank palette
The clean slate
The smooth dance floor
On which to create,
To allow me to listen and
Receive the Wisdom of Life

And all that it has to offer,
Before I think and speak
With clarity, in truth,
From my heart, giving
All that I have to offer Life,

These are my two ways
Of communication,
Of relationship give and take
Speaking and Listening
Energy moving out and Energy coming in
Listening to Speak
Receiving and Giving

-AJA, 02-02-2020

MY SPIRALING SPINE

My eyes look,
my head follows or leads.
They must make that decision together, spiraling,
working as one,
so I can see where I'm going.

My chest rolls with the waves
of my breath.
I isolate to stretch
my spiral flexibility.

I shimmy to shake if off.

I undulate to really feel the
emotion of the music.

Music changes,
beat picks up,
dancey, bright jazz.
Hips sway, then bump to the beat,
pelvic circles,
spiraling oscillations,
swirling waves of bliss.

I remember to care for my
neck and head,
the heavy weight of life,
all the thinking and reasoning,
bending down in despair
or up in hopeful prayer.

I remember to care for my
heart inside that beautifully open,
intricately carved chest chamber.
Hold close
and share with others.

I remember to care for the
delicate crystal bowl
that is my pelvis.
Delicate, but still able to rock on
when the need arises.

I remember to find stillness
from time to time,
for rest, recovery, replenishment,
of my three body weights,
working together as one to heal

AJA, May 2023

MYSTERIES

This Life holds so many mysteries
the answers to which
remain unknown to me…

Why a morning chickadee
speaks directly to me
as if I was his closest confidant.

Why a bi-color rose
makes me hold my gaze
upon it for so long,
wondering how those hues
can split and blend so well,
all the while captivating me with
subtle scents, fresh and sweet.

Why the sounds of tribal drums
captivate me just as much
as the classical strings of an orchestra.

Why my life-long friend,
who held within her quick mind,
more of our childhood memories
than I could…
Who always made me laugh
just by hearing her laugh…
Who makes me regret
the days we never got to share,
because our lives
had other plans for us…
Why she had to go so soon,

from a cancer
that stripped her body's breath
of her life-affirming friendship.

My grief still haunts me
two years out.
Unable to be by her side,
the pandemic in the way
of our last goodbyes.

The mystery of it all haunts me;
and yet, I'm so grateful
for it all...even the regrets,
for it makes me who I am
with the ability to see, feel,
find my strength, and sometimes
understand.
But mostly to appreciate
the mysteries of Life.

–AJA, Oct2022

NEW PERSPECTIVE

I went to ecstatic dance last night
I knew I had to go
even by myself
glad for the opportunity to move
to be free to express
what I've been feeling

But what is it that I've been feeling?

Well I was in tears
even before I arrived at the door
and as I began the slow moves of warming up
awakening my body
I felt a wave
a wave, Gabrielle!!!
a wave of grief
of oppression
of the weight of the world, my world
hanging on me like a dark, heavy cloak

Angular movements took over my body
Jabbing……. poking   lashing
like fingernails sticking and scratching
every part of me

I looked around the room
everyone in the throes of their own worlds
wherever that was
yet experienced altogether
as one writhing, chaotic sea

I gradually realized that my dark,
prickly cloak
was my perception
of my commitments
of my duties
of my feeling of taking care
of everyone else
their burdens were my burdens
their pain was my pain
even if they did not realize it
I felt it deep inside
waiting for release

As the music changed its tune
I changed mine
I knew instinctively
that I could dance my way out
a real life "dancing through life" Nia moment

So I listened
to different parts of the music
high, sweet strings
soft, acoustic guitar
tinkling of bells

There was always something there
telling me another story
giving me another perspective
and a way out of suffering

I needed only to choose to release in freedom
in universal joy and contentment

(With gratitude to Nia®)

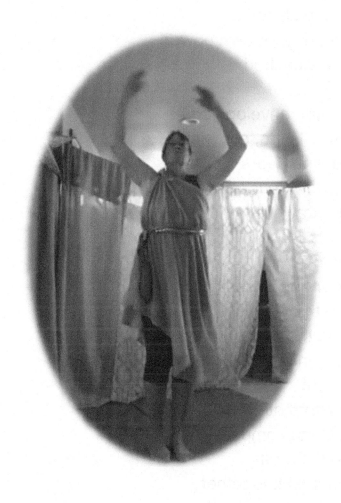

No Strings

Feel your body float
into the earth
letting yourself settle
softly, under your own power
no strings attached

Let the earth envelop you
so you can let go, completely
let go, of your fears
your worries, your attachments
at least for awhile

Breathe in
any anger and despair, and
let it flow through you
down into the earth
where it can be transformed
Breathe out
that transformation
of peace and compassion
you and the earth
in this moment, together
creating and casting off
any leftover strings

Direct your attention
to your resting eyes
your resting mouth
your resting ears
your whole face in quiet release
neck and shoulders release…
…with a sigh of relief
as arms and hands
sink deeper into earth

Give permission to your hips
to rock gently, then release
finding that sweet spot
where they can free their tension
delivering release
down your legs, to your feet
especially your feet
no strings, no tension
just stillness and calm

-AJA, Winter/Spring 2022

Now is Your Moment (FAMSS)

Now…**This**…is your moment!
Breathe this moment in slowly
to your lungs & belly
filling you with calm

Breathe it in
to your shoulders & hips
your arms & legs
your hands & feet
filling you with
strength & stability

For a moment
breathe in and feel the sensation
of flexibility
the long, deep stretches
of your muscles
along your bones

For a moment
breathe in and feel the sensation
of agility
tickling your fingers & toes
and the quick start & stop
of shimmies & hip bumps

For a moment
breathe in and feel the sensation
of mobility
the constant, smooth motion
spine & arms spiraling
hips opening
joints lubricating

Breathe in this moment
to your skin
filling every pore with awareness
allowing it to touch
your connective tissue
to help it do its job
supporting & protecting your body
its strength & stability

Breathe it in to your heart
filling you with unconditional love
for yourself
and everyone around you

Breathe in this moment
and see it with your mind's eye
filling you with light
shining the way along your path

---AJA,4/10/14, 5/10/21

PEACEFUL RENEWAL

How can I accomplish renewal in myself?
How can I continue to grow in a more productive and
creative way?
What will it take?

Perhaps getting rid of old thoughts and baggage from
the past.
Perhaps taking out that baggage/garbage
and recycling it into something new,
something healing for my body and
soul.

Perhaps getting rid of my warring ways,
my us vs. them mentality
my conflicting thoughts and actions

Maybe I can "bury the hatchet" and let peace grow.

Maybe I can find new symbolic meaning
in new thoughts and actions,
and spread peaceful, strength
gestures
like drumbeats and heartbeats
bringing balance and renewal, and practicing self-love.

-AJA, March 2020

REACH OUT YOUR HANDS & FEET & BE A STAR

sense yourself as a star,
radiating from the inside out
to the universe

yes? a tiny speck of a speck
with your own projections,
your interpretations,
your own joys, and fears,
your own journey
but you are so much a part
of the wider whole

just as important
for your contributions,
your being
just as intelligent,
just as beautiful,
your dance
just as necessary

now, hold that universe
in the palms of your hands
and in the center of your heart

you are one with it
that universe
and it with you
one with it
in the center of your soul

— AJA, Jan 12, 2020

RELEASE

Release in your own natural time.

Relax in your own natural time.

Renew in your own natural time.

Breathe in your own natural time

And when you Body is ready,

Arise in your own natural time.

-AJA, May 2019

RELEASE IN YOUR OWN NATURAL TIME

Relax in your own natural time

Renew in your own natural time

Breathe in your own natural time

And when your Body is ready

Arise in your own natural time

...AJA, May 2019

RHYTHM (DANCE CLASS VERSION)

Breathe!
Sense your heart
The beat of your being
The rhythm of your life

Imagine the beat of another's heart
The individual rhythms of others
Surrounding and joining
Separate yet together

Breathe!
Sense the rhythm of the seasons
The feel of the heat
The remembrance of cold and wet
and longing for a cozy, crackling,
rhythmic fire

Sense the anticipation and release
The sweat and joy of today's dance
The beat of the sounds inside your head
The feel of a cool shower coming

Breathe!
Sense your voice
Humming along
The cadence, the tempo
The musical phrase

Sense the rhythm
Even when no drums are beating
No shakers shaking
There is still the ebb and flow
The up and down
The back and forth

Sense the rhythm of life
In your heart
Your own connection
To the rhythm of life

-AJA, Undated

SELF-HEALING

How can I heal myself? Where do I even start?

First of all...
Where is the pain?
Is it in my feet or knees from previous injuries...
sprained ankles or
meniscus tears,
shoulder strains or
back aches,
stiff neck or
migraine?
I can heal from those with help and guidance from
the right source. This I know.

But what of other injuries of the heart and mind... the
weight of the world heavily upon me,
the care of others,
the care for myself
from childhood
and adulthood
traumas?

Some people suffer from outward wars; some of
us from
inner conflicts,
real or imagined.

I must remember
to forgive myself,
for these are not my fault. It is what life gives me to do
with what I can to survive and thrive. I must remember
to forgive myself,
for I cannot cure all. Forgive myself,
and do the best I can to keep breathing
keep living
keep healing myself. It is my sacred work.

– AJA, November 2022

SENSE - ALIGN - CENTER

Sense the earth beneath you
as you relax and breathe.
Notice where your body touches the earth--
the back of your head
the shoulder blades, the sacrum
your calves and heels
the arms and hands---
and the gravity of the earth holding you.

At some point, bend your knees
so that your feet are flat on the floor
and release any lower back pressure.
Be comfortable, and
sense your spine now.
By pushing the heels gently
into the earth, and releasing,
rock the tailbone up & down.
Feel this from the back of your head
to the base of your spine.
Sense that gentle, rocking undulation
up towards the head
and down towards the heels.
A gentle massage of the vertebrae,
the pearls of body connection
from top to bottom and back.
Now relax the spine again,
And using the motion of your heels
and let your hips roll gently side to side,
rocking on the earth, swaying slowly
from right to left, and back again.
The gentle rocking motion reminiscent---

like the pulse of a mother's heartbeat,
of one's own heartbeat,
of the Earth's heartbeat
as you gently sway, up & down, back & forth.

Relax now, and sense your heartbeat
the collective heartbeats of others
pulsing the rhythms of our lives,
of the Earth's life
and the coming of a new season.

Let your body rest, releasing your legs down.
Notice the alignment of spine,
as you lengthen your head and neck,
arms and legs, as they reach out
in all directions like a star.
Sense your Self in the center
of that alignment, that star,
the long bones and short bones.
Then sense Your center of gravity,
the hara, just below the navel.
Notice again your breath,
and a centering into calmness
of Your body, mind, emotions, and spirit.
A calming, healing gift to self
from self, and from the Earth.

-AJA, June 2021

SING

Let's sing…
Sing to our mothers.
Sing to our fathers.
Sing to all who have passed here before
and to all who will come.
Sing to your fellow singers
and sing to yourself
for we are a beauty,
an astonishing mass of feeling
and doing.
Even with our imagined flaws,
they are a beauty too.
For they help us to learn
and grow
and feel
and sing.

AJA, Mother's Day, May 11, 2014

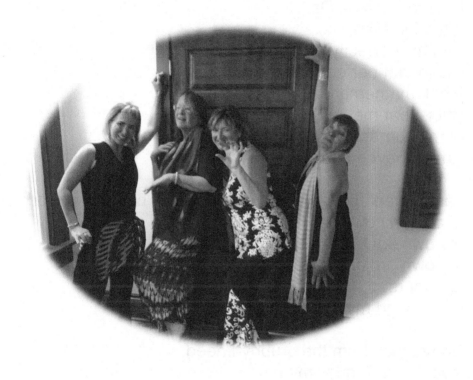

SYMBOLOGY

Shapes in space.
What shape do I project to the world?
What symbol is most characteristic
of me?
I like to imagine Da Vinci's
Vitruvian Man,
with his perfectly proportioned body,
within that perfect circle.
Ideal, mathematical, artistic.
But is that me, my ideal shape
of my human condition?
Hmm, maybe not.

I am not an ideal, mathematical model, but I am a work
of art...my own art,
my own soul,
my own projection of happiness
and fears,
my joy and my well-being.

Sometimes I am the grubby-kneed,
sweaty, dirt-under-my-nails,
hunched-over gardener
tending to my plants.

Sometimes I am the poised dancer
lifting my spine up and out,
relaxing my limbs,
head and eye movements
taking in my surroundings,
waiting for the music to start.

Sometimes I like to let my self imagine
my own body at the center
of an energy field,
much like the electromagnetic field
circling the earth,
top to bottom and back.
I sense myself flowing up and out,
flowing across space,
flowing across time,
sensing the oneness,
sensing all in the universe,
the Yin and Yang of the cosmos.
It's available to all of us
in our collective, connected
symbology.
What is your symbol?

AJA, Feb. 2021

Taking Stock On My 70th Birthday

Recently
I was reminded
to look at my old photos
once in a while
the ones I took
to see what was most important
to me at the time
try to remember the details
try to capture the mood

What I discover
is that most of my photos
are of landscapes,
plants, trees,
things that live on the ground
or fly in the sky,
things of beauty outside of myself.
Not of people.
Why is that?
Am I so afraid of seeing myself,
of seeing others with me?

What happened to me
to make this so?

Was it my childhood experiences
of not wanting to be seen
by others
for whatever reason
they wanted to see me?
Is it because I did not like

what I looked like,
dreaded what others would think?
To this day
I would rather not
have my photo taken,
like it was, that day
by a strange man
in the grocery store.
I guess it reminded me
of the fear I felt
as a child, as a teen trying
to stay out of the limelight.

Will I ever be free of that fear,
that fear of what haunted me
as a child,
but which no longer exists.

-AJA, Jan 9, 2023

THE LAST DANCE - A TRIBUTE TO OUR NIA BODIES

Beginning as a thought, in my tiny, forming brain,
"I want to move!"
Thank you brain, for my thoughts.

Moving from my heart center, giving and receiving love energy,
keeping me going through any situation.
Thank you heart, for my emotions.

Deep in my hara, my center of gravity, helping me balance my body,
through stability and mobility.
Thank you hara, for centering me.

Moving with my legs and feet, the hands that touch the earth,
allowing me to guide and turn and travel in directions.
Thank you feet for your stability and movement.

My arms and hands, flowing or punching, sharp or smooth, flicks or claws,
giving expression to my every move.
Thank you arms and hands for the beauty and the power.

Watching legs moving forward and back,
expressive arms, articulating feet, smiling faces,
through free dance, form and floor work.
Thank you Nia Dancers, for your spirit, your creativity,
your passion, your love.

It has been an honor for me to share Nia with you, this
first year of teaching.

AJA, Date Unknown

THE RHYTHM OF THE DANCE ARTS

Sense the dance of your heart the beat of
your being the rhythm of your life

Imagine the beat of another's heart the
individual rhythms of others surrounding and
joining separate yet together

Sense the rhythm of the seasons the feel of
the heat coming
the remembrance of cold and wet and
longing for a cozy, crackling rhythmic fire

Remember the rhythm of Jazz dance in your
body
syncopated, hip bumps, flash of hands fun,
showy, sensual

Remember the style of Modern Dance the
contraction and release emotionally charged
inward then outward
shapes in space

Remember the energy of Duncan Dance sweet
flowing, free-spirited up in the air, then
grounded to the earth
sometimes tragic
other times completely ecstatic

Sense the anticipation and release the sweat
of today's dance the rhythm of the sounds
slowly retreating
the feel of a cleansing shower to come

Sense the rhythm, now
even when no drums are beating no
shakers shaking

There is still the flow of breath in the
silences
in the quiet, between
the notes of birds and bells in the wind

Come back to your heart
your beat and the quiet in between
and sense your connection
to the rhythm of life
within your own dance

AJA May 2021

THE UPPERS

I sense my hands,
the beautifully aged fingertips and
palms, arthritic joints and all. They've
done so much for me. I'm so grateful
for my hands.
I can feed myself and write a letter,
brush my hair, clap the beat, and start
seeds of tomatoes and
peas.

My arms being connected
to my hands,
allow emotional expression
or put up a good fight -
blocking, punching,
striking whatever might hinder
my existence,
metaphorically or otherwise.
My arms allow mobility, agility,
and the sensation of strength.

My shoulders have held so much
during my life and shrugged off what
does not serve me, letting my heart
open and letting me stand tall.

My shoulders
have done so much work
engaging muscles
of upper back and chest
to lift arms upward
to touch a lilac,
or lift a shovel to dig the garden.
I love the look of a dancing back -
strong, supple, mobile and stable.

Together my upper extremities -
back, shoulders, arms and hands
can lift, twist,
reach down to the earth
and up to the sky.
Touch the water
and feel the warmth of fire.

I am so grateful for their movements,
their strengths and weaknesses
reminding me to keep
working it out.

-AJA, June, 2021

THIS RHYTHM OF LIFE

This rhythm of Life
is our birthright
we share it with all things
insects and kings
Humming and beating
swaying and stomping
pulsing hearts
a dance of art
This rhythm of Life
gives the gift of Seasons
and reasons
to keep on breathin' on
Hot summer
lake shimmers
turning leaves
colors weave
rain and thunder
awash with wonder
The white of winter
cold and bitter, and
blissful, frosted,
beauty scenes
And later, to spring
newness brings
seeds of life
all is right

Rhythm rules

-AJA 2018, 2023

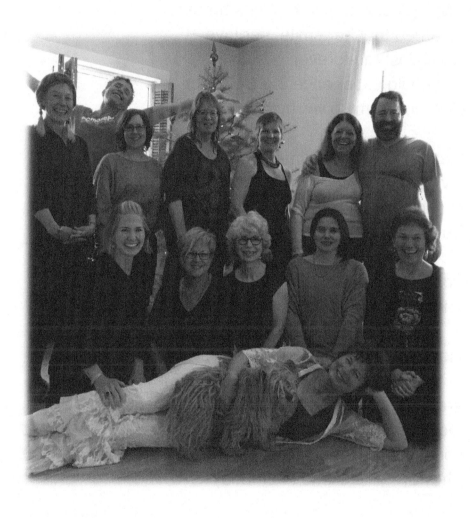

Trust *(Form & Freedom in the Dance of Life)*

I learned how to trust when I was young,
holding softly to my mother's breast.
I learned that her smile, her love
would last me forever
so I could experience the **freedom**
to dance to my own rhythm.

I learned that sometimes, though
love and trust can be broken,
causing chaos, arguments, breakups.
But I learned that love and trust
would come again, maybe in another **form**
from another being, another source,
another way to dance, restoring my flow.

I learned later in life to really trust myself…
to trust **that all that happens** to me
are lessons life gives to me,
the cruelties and mercies,
complacencies and compassions.
They are all lessons to embody.

But it's not just about me
and my little slice of life.
It's about the wholeness of existence
the yin and yang of life,
giving me all the **forms** to experience

the steps and stances, and other life lessons
as well as the **freedom** to think, feel,
express, and trust my own dance.

May we look to our Mother, Nature,
follow her lead,
trust and embrace the **forms**,
love and respect our **freedoms.**
Choose to dance with her
embracing the two sides
so a new way of living can arise
with responsibility to one another,

- one with no need of judgment
- one where all beings radiate harmony
- one where the seemingly opposite forces of yin
  and yang coexist,

as they **do** in Nature, balancing
and complimenting each other…
trusting, loving and taking care
of each other
Think of the possibilities.

-AJA, Nov 3, 2021

SOLITARY OR SURROUNDED

Sometimes it's challenging
to sense my own rhythm;
when to work, when to play
when to just sit
and let my mind wander
aimlessly, or totally empty.

I love being surrounded by
family and friends;
perhaps you could say
I took over the mothering job,
(as many of us do)
after mine passed,
even though
I'm not the eldest.

But I am the one
who has surrendered herself
to that task.

I love my family and friends
and would do anything
in my power to help them
however I can.

But sometimes
I just need my Self
to reflect on my health,
my happiness, on the part I play
in this world.
Sometimes,
I need my own mothering,
nurturing, centering,
kiss the boo boo on the head
healing.

I'm so glad that I am learning
to do that for myself,
as well as for others.

Let's take care to listen
to our own Body's Way,
sense our own rhythms,
when to move and groove,
when to rest in solitude,
when to heal.

-AJA, May 2023

this is just how it's supposed to
be

 wondering when and
if
I'll ever get to see you again
to hold you
to laugh and smile with you
share a drink with you
and some yummy dessert

wondering when and
if
I'll ever again feel safe enough
to walk along a beach
on a warm, sunny day
wandering by myself
without a care

wondering when and
if
I can ever again
explore a street full of shops
full of smiling people
talking and laughing with them
shaking their hands
have a nice day
glad to meet you
normal
everyday conversations
and pleasantries

wondering when and
if
a pandemic and a crazed world would
change us so much
that life as we knew it before
never comes back
our relationships drowning
in the overflowing emptiness

wondering when and
if
I could ever get used to a life
of solitude
turning inside
listening to the inner voice
that perhaps has more to tell me
than I ever dreamed possible
about life
about sensing my tiny
but essential
place in the grand scheme
about the web of life
in all its intricacies
accomplishments
and desperations

what if
turning deep inside
is just how I'm supposed to
be   -AJA, Date Unknown

WHEN I DANCE

I feel so young again

I feel like I did
Before all those rules
Were put upon me as a child

"Be this way"
"Don't do that way"
"Quiet your voice"
"Don't make noise"
"Sit still"
"Don't act weird"

When I dance
I can go back again
To being free
To move
To squeal
To clap
To cry
To laugh
And cry again with Joy

When I dance
I return
To the primal good in me
And whatever I'm connected to
Whatever comes into my life
From before
From my ancestors
From the animals
From the trees
From the earth
From the stars

When I dance
It is a gift I give
To myself
And share with the world

When I dance
My soul is opened up
My body moves in wider circles
My life makes sense again

-AJA, Date Unknown

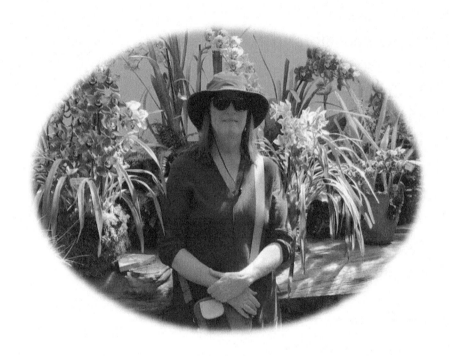

Made in the USA
Monee, IL
13 September 2024

65210271R00072